Punk Azz Cancer, How Dare You!

This book is dedicated to my amazing husband Roman, with him, my life has no limits; to my beautiful babies Rhylei and Rhoen, you have given me unspeakable joy and immeasurable happiness; to my family: Lakora, Lionel, Errol Sr., Brana and Errol Jr., thank you for your unconditional love and support; and to Dr. H. C. Kinley, my mentor, without you, none of this would be possible.

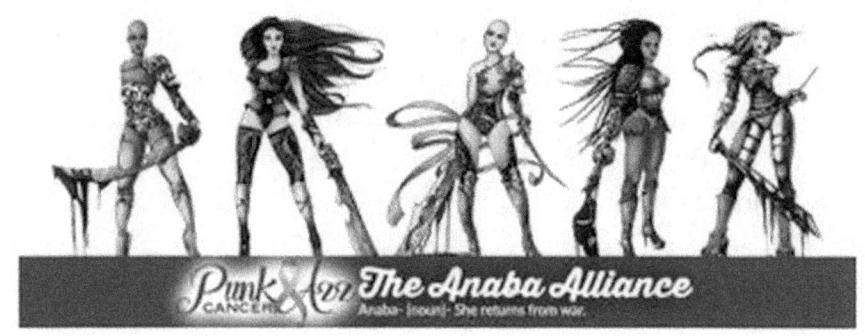

Visit punkazzcancer.com for Breast Cancer
resources and Anaba Alliance merchandise and apparel.

Punk azz cancer sucker-punched me in the gut. That's exactly what it felt like. I was shocked and embarrassed. How could I be fabulous with breast cancer? Right? Where's the power in being sick? Cancer took away my badazzness. And for a while, I lived in a darkness so thick I could touch it. Breast cancer introduced me to a level of fear I never imagined I would ever experience. I became depressed and reclusive. I felt devastated, defeated, and at times inconsolable.

I hardly recognized the frightened woman in the mirror. She was not me. I could handle anything. Couldn't I? It was difficult to accept her as the new me - a broken me, a terrified me. I guess I wasn't that brave after all........

OR SO I THOUGHT.

In the midst of tragedy, we feel hopeless. We are surrounded by darkness and despair. It's not that we lack power; it's that we lack the awareness of it and we lack the belief in it. When we tap into our personal power, we learn to become resilient. And soon, we become completely unfazed by the very same things that would have previously forced us to our knees. Over time, I was able to overcome that fear and reclaim my power. It is my hope that, through this book, you are inspired to reclaim your power as well.

My dark days gave me a story, they didn't make me powerful. I was already powerful- so are you.

Believe it.

TABLE OF CONTENTS

Cancer Is A Punk

The dictionary describes a "punk" as a cowardly or weak individual. In many communities the term "punk" is used to describe a person who sneaks up on you and attacks you when you least expect it. A punk sucker-punches you when you are not prepared. A punk takes you down without giving you any warning. Cancer is *definitely* a punk.

I have never been a punk. I have always had a courageous personality, not easily scared, not easily intimidated. I was Sly Fox, the owner of and head investigator at Sly Fox Investigations, an all-female investigative agency that I personally grew from a company with zero dollars to a six-figure brand—with two babies on my hips! I was a visionary, a leader, a female entrepreneur, a sassy combination of brains, beauty, and boss. I was sailing full steam ahead toward all my dreams. I found the greatest pleasure in accomplishing each one of them.

My biggest accomplishment was my success with my private investigation agency. Private investigation is a hugely male-dominated industry. There are approximately sixty thousand PIs in the United States today; only 15 percent are women, and only 3 percent of those are African American women. I took pride in the fact that I was able to make my mark in an industry where, at times, I wasn't always welcomed with open arms. I became a nationally recognized investigator. I was featured in such publications as *Essence* magazine, *225* magazine, the *Baton Rouge Business Report*, the *Atlanta Post*, and many more. I would get calls every year from production companies that wanted to create TV shows around my brand and my team. I was even previously appointed the director of Region II of the Louisiana Private Investigators Association.

I wanted it all. I wholeheartedly rejected the notion that women cannot be successful in business and still raise a family. Society tells us that we have to choose one or the other; I never bought into that notion. I was not only a businesswoman but also a woman with an amazing husband and two toddlers.

Life was good. Little did I know, however, that my world would be turned upside down with one phone call.

The Call

On a beautiful afternoon, I was driving to my office, my two babies in the backseat, the sunroof open, the warm sun shining down on our faces. We were jamming! My babies and I were singing a version of "The Wheels on the Bus" (you know, they go round and round, round and round) that would put any *American Idol* contestant to shame. That moment with my girl and my boy could not have been more perfect. As I was pulling into the parking lot of my office, I heard my phone ring. I started gesturing to the children to lower their voices so I could hear, because they were in full-fledged concert mode at that time.

"Hello? Yes, this is Brianne." It was my doctor. "Yes. I'm sorry about the noise," I said as I laughed. "My kids are having a concert. Let me step outside so I can hear you a little bit better." I stepped out of my car. "Yes, Doctor, what is it that you're trying to tell me?"

"We received your biopsy reports, and I'm sorry to tell you that you have breast cancer."

"Breast cancer? Well, there must be some mistake," I said. "Nobody in my family has breast cancer. Nobody. There's no family history of breast cancer with anyone. I'm only in my thirties; how is this even possible?"

"I'm sorry, but you do have breast cancer, and I'm going to refer you to a breast cancer surgeon so that we can discuss your next steps."

I hung up the phone, and my environment grew quiet as I stared straight ahead in disbelief. I heard nothing; my ears would not work. I saw a redbird singing on the fence nearby, yet his song was silent. I saw his beak open and close, yet there was no sound. The earth stopped. I could no longer feel my body; the air felt thick, and it became difficult to fill my lungs. I was paralyzed. I stopped breathing. In the midst of the silence, the only sound I could hear was my heart thumping inside my chest louder and louder, faster and faster. I was panicking internally. I was suffocating in fear. I felt the burning sensation of my eyes welling up with tears. I continued to stare ahead, standing stiff as a statue in a moment completely void of sound.

Slowly I began to hear a faint banging noise coming from car, and slowly I turned my head toward the sound. It was my daughter, Rhylei, banging on the car window, trying to get my attention. As soon as I made eye contact with her, the air reentered my lungs, and I gasped quickly and forcefully like a drowning child who has just grasped his first breath of air above water. I was back. Although I could hear again, I still could not feel the earth under my feet. My legs were numb. I slowly walked to my car door using the car as a crutch, walking ever so slowly along the side of my car, holding myself up with my left arm, afraid to let go and fall into the unknown.

I leaned my back against the door and called my husband. When he answered I whispered, "They said I have cancer." I remember speaking very slowly and quietly, as if I had a secret I didn't really want to share. When I said the words, I felt as if the words came from an external source, as if someone else was breaking the news to my husband and to me at the same time.

I felt the same amount of shock as he did when he yelled, "What?" "Cancer?"

My eyes welled up with tears, and in a monotone voice, I continued to speak. "The doctor said he doesn't know much about the cancer yet. He only knows it's cancer. I have to see a specialist."

"Are they sure?" my husband asked.

I was silent.

"Hello? Are they sure?" he asked again.

More silence. Words escaped me. My heart thumped harder and harder again; my breath became rapid, and then I let out a high-pitched, muffled squeal. I was screaming without screaming. I was screaming without opening my mouth so as not to upset my babies who were watching and listening. All I could do was scream—hysterically, emotionally, internally. My husband said, "Breathe, bae. You're going to be fine. Just breathe." I took a deep breath and told him I would call him back.

I hung up the phone, looked at my babies, smiled, wiped my tears, and said, "Let's go to Mawmaw's house."

Unimaginable Reality

I dialed my mom's number as I was driving out of the parking lot. When she answered, I told her, "They said I have breast cancer. I have my kids with me. I can't breathe. Can we come over there?"

And in a calm and reassuring voice, my mom said, "Yes, it's OK; you're going to be OK. Come over here now."

I hung up, called my cousin and best friend, Nicol, and told her the news. She said, "I don't believe that; I don't believe that shit. No, you don't. You don't have breast cancer."

As the tears rolled down my cheeks, I said, "I do. I do, Nicol. That's what they told me."

She said, "Stop driving. You're in no condition to drive."

Nicol was far away in California; she was always a straight, no-chaser type of chick. She was always very blunt and always spoke her mind. Nicol always told me the truth, and there was nothing more I wanted in the world than for her words to be true that day. I did not want breast cancer. I really wished she were closer because I knew I needed her reassurance. I knew I needed her strength because I could definitely feel mine slipping away.

I received that dreadful phone call on a Thursday afternoon. The earliest appointment I could get was the next Tuesday. So from Thursday to Tuesday, I had no information about the extent of my breast cancer. For a while I was left with only my own preconceived notions and thoughts about cancer. I knew nothing about cancer. The only thing I knew was that it can kill you. The gravity of my thoughts sent me completely over the edge. I had no idea how I got this disease. How did I get this? Was it something I ate? Something I didn't eat? I decided to Google "breast cancer" for more information—and that's the one thing I now advise newly diagnosed people *never to do*. I looked it up on the Internet. And, in an innocent attempt to educate myself, I inadvertently diagnosed myself with every worst-case breast cancer scenario the Internet had to offer. Instant panic ensued. OMG! I gave myself the rarest form of incurable cancer known to man, and it completely freaked me out. I searched for answers and cures and medications online. I searched for someone, anyone, who could tell me whether or not I was about to die. More panic set in. I finally found a breast cancer forum online, and I told everyone what I discovered on the Internet, and everyone in the forum had the same response: Log off! Get off the Internet!

If you are newly diagnosed, do yourself a favor and wait until you talk to your doctor. Do not try to figure this out yourself. You'll only get more upset and confused and...if you're like me...depressed.

How Dare You!

The thought of my babies being without their mother sucked the life from my existence; the pain in my chest was so heavy it anchored me to the floor daily. Life without my babies was the equivalent of death to me. Life without my husband was unspeakable. There was no life for me without them. I was terrified at the thought of dying while my babies were still young. As an adult right now, I couldn't remember anything I did when I was three years old, let alone one year old. If something happened to me now, would my babies forget me? Would they even know who I was? I grabbed my son, Rhoen, as he waddled past me. I hugged him so tightly that he said, "Mommy, let go!"

"No," I said. I wanted to smell him. I sniffed his hair long and hard; I smelled his neck and his arms as he struggled to get away. I needed to breathe him into me so I could recall his scent whenever I needed to. Finally he broke free and ran off, looking back at me as if I was crazy or deranged. I watched him run away. The sunlight captured his golden curly hair shining like a crown on his head; he was royalty to me—a prince, my sweet baby boy—so beautiful, so sweet. How could I not be around to watch him grow up? I imagined him at seven years old, fourteen years old, at twenty-one. How could I not be there? How is my not being there even a possibility? Before my diagnosis, this would have been unfathomable; now it was a real possibility—a possibility that took me to a very dark place, mentally and emotionally.

And what about my sweet baby girl, Rhylei? Her hair so soft, curly, and full. She was born with a full head of hair. She was the first newborn I had ever seen in my life who looked like she was wearing a wig. Now, at three years old, her hair was hanging to right above her butt. Gorgeous baby girl—so intelligent, smart,

8

and bossy. A leader. Telling everybody what to do. My kind of girl. How could I not be around to watch my beautiful princess find her feet in the world? Who was going to comb her hair? Who would plan her sweet-sixteen party? Who would take her shopping for her first bra? How dare this dumb azz disease try to take me away from my babies? Would my husband remarry? Would some strange woman claim my daughter as her own? I felt the panic set in again as I contemplated all these questions. No, I decided. No strange woman will ever take my place. That bitch better not try. Whoever she was, she'd better stay away from my babies. I told my husband that if I died he'd better not remarry, because I would haunt the house until she left. She could never be me. I was enraged at the very thought of my husband being with someone else. "I'm serious, Roman," I said. "I'm going to haunt your azz, and I'm going to haunt her azz too."

He smiled and said, "Bae, what are you talking about? You're not going anywhere."

"I'm just saying," I answered. "If."

Now, as selfish as that may sound, that was my immediate first reaction to the idea of someone else raising my children. I wasn't ready or willing to share them.

What about my husband? My husband is the most amazing man in the world. Our life together is nothing short of a beautiful love story. My husband is intelligent, sweet, sexy, smooth, strong, and hilarious—a gift from heaven. I could not imagine life without him. I could not imagine experiencing breast cancer without him by my side. I'm always comforted in his arms, and I feel safe when he is near. He's my biggest fan, my biggest supporter, and my best friend. I recall the moment that undoubtedly assured me of just how deep our connection was—just how much this amazing man truly loved me. It is a moment I will never forget. I was crying hysterically one day shortly after I received my diagnosis. I was engulfed in fear, and I was feeling defeated, hopeless, and terrified. My husband held me tightly as I wept, his shirt becoming more and more soaked with tears as I buried my face deeper and deeper into his chest. "I can't do this," I said. "Oh my God, I have cancer! I can't do this!" I screamed.

My husband pulled me away from his chest, slowly lifted my chin, and stared into my eyes. He spoke very slowly as if my life depended on the words he was about to speak.

"I have cancer, bae," I said.

He shook his head no, wiped my tears, and said, "No. No. *You* don't have cancer, bae. You don't have cancer. *We* have cancer. This is not your fight. This is *our* fight. We have cancer."

That very moment changed my entire perspective. In that very moment, I realized just how much this man loved me. I knew in my heart that if I died that night, I would die feeling completely loved and adored. Cancer can take a lot of things away, but it cannot touch love.

Wasting Away

Imagine staring into pitch-black darkness. A darkness so thick you can reach out and touch it. Darkness became an unhealthy safe haven for me. I became really depressed after my breast cancer diagnosis. I was so depressed my doctors prescribed Prozac to help me deal with what I was experiencing. I couldn't eat; I couldn't sleep; I couldn't move. For weeks I was bedridden; I wanted to get up, but I just physically could not move. My family, concerned about my mental health, kept a watchful eye on me. They felt it. They knew that this diagnosis had sucker-punched me right in the gut. It took my spunk, it took my voice, and it took my power- my lift energy, my desire to move forward. I lost my ambition. I lost my drive. I felt completely hopeless.

I could see my family talking to me, but I could not comprehend anything they were saying; I was in another world. And for the moment, I could not recall any stories of people beating cancer. All I could recall were stories of people who had died from cancer. In my mind, I was going to die from cancer, and I literally could not come to grips with such a reality. It was too much. One day you're laughing, smiling, and loving life; the next day, you're facing your mortality, wondering just how long you have left to live? I became reclusive as I hid inside the darkness. To me, darkness was comforting. Light only confirmed my painful reality.

For a while I remained in my powerless stupor. I wasn't eating. I wasn't drinking. I wanted to waste away, and my haggard face and lack of energy showed it. I didn't want to fight. I didn't want to be a member of the breast cancer club. I had no concern for my physical appearance. I was mentally immobile. Paralyzed. I couldn't wake up from this terrible nightmare. I was shocked, disbelieving, and embarrassed. How can I be fabulous with breast cancer? I mean, the Sly Fox was fabulous, wasn't she? Where's the swag in having breast cancer? Cancer had taken away my badazzness. In my mind, people would always look at me as sick. Where is the power in being sick? I thought. Cancer was taking away my strength. Prior to my diagnosis, I would effortlessly dive into opportunities far outside of my comfort zone. I was brave. I was bold. I used to be courageous. Used to be. Prior to my diagnosis, I loved to inspire and encourage those around me to pursue their dreams and to aspire to be great. People valued my advice and looked to me for guidance on entrepreneurship. I tried to use my voice to affect people positively every day. Cancer took that desire away from me. I lost my voice; it was lost in the darkness.

After a while my mom decided enough was enough. She knew how dangerous it was for me to keep flirting with depression, so one Saturday afternoon she came to my house with a lunch she had prepared. I, of course, was still in bed in the dark. She came into my bedroom and opened the blinds; the bright sun illuminated the room. She snatched the covers off my face and said, "Get up."

Startled, I protested "Close the blinds, Mom. I don't want to get up!"

She continued to pull the covers completely off of me and said, "No, you are getting out of this bed right now, and we're going to leave this house. You are getting out of this house today. Your babies need you; your husband needs you; you have to get up, and you have to fight."

My babies, my beautiful babies, and my loving husband. Yes, they did need me. They needed me to be strong. I needed to be strong. Suddenly I felt a rush of heat in my body as I was overcome with anger. Look at me! Look at what I've been reduced to! How dare you, cancer! How dare you try to take me away from my kids! How dare you try to take me away from my husband! How dare you! My face felt hotter than the sun beaming down on my pillow. I sat on the edge of the bed staring at the wall with such great intensity in my eyes as if trying to suppress my overwhelming desire to punch the wall, punch the desk, punch anything. Cancer became an entity to me in that moment—a person I wanted to punch in the face, someone I needed to take revenge on for sucker punching me in the gut like a punk. As I rose up out of the bed, I mumbled in disgust, "Punk azz cancer," and walked to the bathroom to wash my face.

I found out I had stage zero and stage one breast cancer. I was diagnosed with invasive ductal carcinoma (IDC) and ductal carcinoma in situ (DCIS), and I was scheduled to have a lumpectomy to remove the cancerous tumor.

On the morning of my surgery, my alarm clock chimed at 4:00 a.m. Today was the day. I was having a lumpectomy. I had mixed feelings about it. I was happy that I was getting rid of the deadly invasive tumor, yet I was sad that my breasts would have to be mutilated in the process. I let out a deep sigh. A moment later, I felt my husband's hand on my thigh; he knew what I was feeling and with one simple gesture, even in his sleep, he tried to reassure me that everything would be OK. I got out of bed, went into the bathroom, and turned the shower on. I stood in the shower with my eyes closed as the warm water rolled down my face to my neck, and down to my breast. I looked down at my breasts and smiled. They were beautiful to me. My girls: Thelma and Louise.

I thought about how my breasts nurtured my babies when I breastfed them. I smiled as I remembered the feeling of my babies suckling my breasts as I gave them nourishment. I cupped both of my breasts in the palms of my hands, closed my eyes, and gave them a gentle squeeze. I was proud of my boobs. I thought I had a nice rack. They were perfect to me. I smiled again, basking in a moment of undeniable breast awesomeness. Then, in a strange moment of realization, I snatched my hands from my breasts. Oh my God, my breasts are trying to kill me! What the hell! I was pissed again. Stupid azz breasts, I thought. I cupped my left breast, Thelma; she was good in my book; she wasn't trying to kill me. But that right breast, Louise? That bitch had to go.

When I got out of the steamy shower, I stood quietly in front of the sink, staring into the foggy mirror that showed no reflection due to the steam. Time stood still for a moment. It was eerie and surreal. I felt like I was in a foggy graveyard in a different world—a dreadful place where death was imminent. Not the death of me entirely, but the death of a piece of me, a piece of my soul. I think my mind was preparing me for the imminent loss I was about to experience. Tears rolled down my face. I didn't want to have to do this; why did I have to have breast cancer? Why me? I didn't understand. My chest hurt. I felt my heart rate increasing. Would I die soon? How long did I really have to live? Were my doctors telling me everything? More tears flowed as I was bombarded with all these questions.

A knock on the bathroom door startled me back into reality; then I heard my husband's voice, "Bae, are you all right in there?"

I quickly grabbed my towel, wiped my tears, cleared my throat, and said, "Yes, bae, I'm fine. I'll be out in a second." I slowly raised my hand, and in one smooth motion, I wiped a little steam from the mirror. I could see only my eyes. I stared into my eyes for a moment, hardly recognizing the terrified woman staring back at me. I closed my eyes quickly and forcefully, trying hard to erase the image of the woman I just saw. She was not me. I was brave, wasn't I? I could handle anything, couldn't I? It was difficult for me to accept her as the new "me"—a new, terrified me. A me whose light had been dimmed. I guess I wasn't that brave after all....

When I came out of the bathroom, I walked to my closet to get dressed: a T-shirt and sweat pants, the usual. When people say you wear what you feel, they're right. I had become frumpy Felicia. I felt dreadful and dreary on the inside, so I wore dreadful and dreary clothes on the outside. I had no desire to dress up. There was no need to dress up when my spirits were down. As I was about to slip into my usual dreary uniform, I paused for a minute, realizing again just how much my breasts would never look the same once I left the house today. My breasts would never look the same. Wow. I shivered at the thought. I ran over to my dresser and started digging through my lingerie drawer; oh my God, I won't look right in any of this anymore! I looked at the time. We had only a few minutes before we needed to leave the house. I looked back into the drawer and quickly pulled out my favorite lingerie. It was a black-lace and rose-colored French-maid outfit that fit perfectly. I felt so pretty in it. I felt sexy in it. I quickly put it on. Oh my God, my breast will never look like this again! Where is my camera? I wanted to take a picture of my pretty boobs in my favorite lingerie before they were sliced up from surgery. I grabbed my cell phone and started taking selfies, smiling, trying to hold on to the moment, trying to hold on to the feeling of seeing my boobs so perfect. It felt good.

As I looked into my camera's lens, about to snap another picture, I noticed the purple-marker lines my doctor had drawn on my breast the previous day. The lines indicated where he intended to cut me during surgery. My heart dropped. I suddenly felt ugly. No more pictures for me. I put the camera down. As I walked across the room to put my camera back in my purse, my husband walked out of the bathroom. He laughed and said, "Bae, what are you doing? Is that what you're wearing to the hospital? Lingerie?"

I laughed. "No! I was just taking pictures so I could remember what my breasts looked like before surgery."

"Let me take some pictures of you."

Remembering my purple-marker lines, I said, "No, that's OK. I took some already."

Sensing my hesitation he smiled and said, "Who's the better photographer? You or I?" I looked down toward the floor, feeling embarrassed and self-conscious. He grabbed my camera and said, "Pose."

"Pose?" I asked.

"Yes, pose. Pose on the bed; pose against the wall; pose everywhere."

"But I have these purple-marker lines—"

He cut me off. "You're beautiful, bae. Just pose." So I did. I posed and smiled and laughed for my entire mini–photo shoot. When we finished, my husband said, "You're beautiful today, tomorrow, and forever." Then he kissed me on the forehead, and I felt my purple-marker lines disappear.

Rap Battle At 5 a.m.

During the ride to the hospital, I was quiet and contemplative, silently watching the cars speed by us on the interstate. The air was crisp and cool. We pulled into the hospital parking lot.

"Are you ready?" my husband asked.

"Nope. I'm not going in."

He laughed. "Yes, you are." He grabbed my hand and gave it a little squeeze.

I closed my eyes and received the calming energy he released to me through his touch. "I need answers. How the hell did I get cancer?" I asked.

"You need answers?" He started scrolling through his cell phone. The next thing I knew the rapper Lil Boosie was blasting from the phone's speakers. I heard Lil Boosie rapping, "I need answers, Lord; tell me why I got cancer."

I laughed hysterically and said, "Oh my God, you've got to be kidding me! Are you seriously playing Lil Boosie before I go into surgery?" Ignoring me, Roman started rapping along with Lil Boosie, dancing in his seat. I laughed and joined in. Now here we were, sitting in the hospital parking lot at 5:00 a.m., rapping and dancing to Lil Boosie right before my lumpectomy. It became a rap battle- who could rap the most enthusiastically. It was hilarious and completely characteristic of the magical way my husband is always able to turn a situation around. I exited the car with a smile on my face. We quickly entered the hospital and got on the elevator that was full of people. My husband started humming Lil Boosie under his breath. I burst out laughing again as we entered the surgery area.

Worst Surprise Ever

The surgery was a success. The doctors removed my cancerous lump; now we just needed to wait for them to call us after the margins were tested. Doctors test the margins of cancer to make sure they got all the disease out and ensure the cancer had not spread to my lymph nodes. If the cancer hadn't spread to my lymph nodes, it meant the cancer had a very low chance of spreading to the rest of my body. This phone call would determine not only how aggressive the tumor was but also whether or not I would need chemotherapy, radiation, or both.

My entire family and I held our breath for an entire week. After a week, my doctor called and got straight to the point. Good news: your cancer has not spread to your lymph nodes; your lymph nodes are completely void of cancer. This means your cancer is contained in your breasts. Oh my God, really? I started crying tears of joy. More good news: your cancer is confirmed to be very small; you caught it early; you don't need chemo, and you probably don't need radiation. Oh my God, really? I screamed with excitement. Bad news: your margins are not clear; we did not get all the cancer out. The DCIS cancer is so widespread in your breast that we recommend a mastectomy.

"What?" I said as I felt my body go limp. "A mastectomy?" You didn't get it all out? What?" He repeated his explanation and advised me to come in to discuss my options. Un-freakin'-believable.

A mastectomy is a procedure where a breast is removed from the body. Some women elect to have their breast reconstructed; some do not. Either way, it's a major surgery. I had a hard time understanding why I had to have a mastectomy for such a small tumor. But my MRI image explained it. The entire right side of my breast was filled with stage-zero precancerous cells; there was no way they could save my breast. I had to lose it.

Looking For Answers

In the weeks preceding my mastectomy, I was completely overwhelmed. My breasts made me a woman, right? I felt like I was going to lose a part of my womanhood. I felt like I would be frowned upon by society—like society would always perceive me as "less than." I needed help; I needed someone to talk to, someone who knew exactly what I was experiencing. I rummaged through my hospital papers and found an address for a cancer services center and immediately drove over. As I pulled into the cancer services center's parking lot, my heart immediately began to race. What if someone I knew saw me here? I became flushed with embarrassment. I looked around frantically trying to identify a familiar vehicle so I could speed out of the parking lot before I was identified. No familiar vehicles were in sight. Whew! That was close. I closed my eyes as I hugged my steering wheel. I imagined, for a moment, that the steering wheeled hugged me back. I needed a hug desperately. I needed to hear that I was not alone. I needed to see others just like me—other young women. Were there any other entrepreneurs here with breast cancer? I wondered. Any businesswomen with breast cancer? Any mothers with breast cancer? Where were these women? How were they dealing with this? I needed answers.

I knew the answers were possibly in that cancer services building—if I could only summon the courage to walk in. I took a deep breath. What the hell was I doing here? I thought. I was about to walk into a cancer services building—not to help a friend or relative but to help myself. I was at a cancer services building for me. I was here for me. Wow. I closed my eyes, forcefully trying to "unhear" my own thoughts. How did I end up here? My eyes stung from the tears welling up. No, Brianne, you cannot cry! You will not cry! Pull yourself together! I took another deep breath, opened my car door, and walked toward the building.

When I entered the building, I saw an old woman standing inside. I smiled and said, "Hi, I'm here for the breast-cancer support group." The room smelled of peppermint and rubbing alcohol. The room was filled with books; it reminded me of a library. An older black female sitting at the desk smiled and said, "It's upstairs on your left."

"Thank you," I replied as I wondered if she also had breast cancer. My legs felt like they weighed thirty pounds each as I ascended the stairs. I ascended very slowly, contemplating whether or not I should just go back home. Run now, Bri. Go get back in the car; it's not too late. Go. No, I was here now. Just keep walking, keep going; you need help, just keep walking. I walked into the room. The meeting had already started. Everyone was sitting at a circular desk eating sandwiches and other lunch food while one woman spoke to the attendees. I walked in with my head down, intentionally trying not to make eye contact with anyone. Once settled in my seat, I slowly raised my head and immediately realized I was the only young person in the room. Where were all the young people? I thought. The room was filled with women who were much older than me. I felt completely out of place, and I wanted to run back out the door. Oh wait, I could see a younger lady sitting at the table. She smiled at me; I smiled back feeling really relieved to see her.

The woman who was addressing the group was explaining an exercise she wanted us to do. She wanted us to write down some of the things we were most proud of prior to our breast cancer diagnosis. I started to write down my accomplishments: owned my own agency, nationally recognized, blah, blah, blah. I smiled as I remembered just how ambitious I was. I wondered if I'd ever feel such ambition again. After we wrote down our accomplishments, everyone took turns sharing them with the group. The woman next to me spoke about her diagnosis, and then said she was most proud of her garden and her grandchildren. I was next. With all eyes on me, I froze. The instructor smiled at me and said, "You don't have to speak if you don't want to." I felt my eyes well up with tears. I fought hard not to cry. Be brave, dammit; be brave in here. Don't you dare cry right now; be brave, I said to myself. My teeth were chattering inside my mouth. My heart raced. Get a hold of yourself, I commanded. Someone handed me a tissue—she had noticed my anxiety.

I took a deep breath, introduced myself, and told everyone when I had been diagnosed. I spoke slowly, trying desperately to remain in control of my voice. I spoke about the type of cancer I had, my accomplishments, and how much my life had changed. I explained my fear and my sadness. I talked and talked and talked—probably too much, more than everyone else for sure. It felt good; it was the first time I had spoken about my breast cancer out loud to a group of strangers. I felt relieved to rid my heart of all the heaviness, embarrassment, and shame. I felt lighter; I felt free—a little. In closing I said that, ultimately, I felt like breast cancer sucker punched me in the gut and silenced me and that I wanted to be my old self again. My eyes immediately stung with tears; saying that out loud felt way too real to me. I felt that in my soul, and it struck me like a bolt of lightning; the truthfulness of that statement was a reality I wasn't ready to face. I started crying inconsolably.

Three of the women rushed over to me. They surrounded me and hugged me at the same time. Each one of them took turns attempting to reassure me that everything would be OK. One of them, an older black woman, said, "Darling, you will find your voice again, and when you do, you will be an amazing testimony to others. Give me your phone number. I want to keep in touch with you. You will do amazing things again, you'll see.

I know you will." At that moment I really didn't want to give her my number because I still didn't believe I belonged there. I gave it to her anyway because I appreciated her kind words. As everyone started walking back to their seats, I felt good that they were so supportive, yet I was embarrassed that I was such a freaking crybaby. I mean, seriously, Brianne, you did the ugly cry in front of all these women, but you don't want people to stare at you? As I took my seat, someone passed me a cookie. I smiled and took a bite. That's right, I thought—a cookie for the crybaby.

As the women continued to go around the circle telling stories, I noticed it was the other young woman's turn to speak. I perked up, eagerly anticipating her story. How old was she? Did she have kids? Did we share the same type of cancer? I immediately claimed her as my new BFF-cancer friend. She smiled at everyone and started to speak.

"Hi, everyone," she began. "I am a volunteer here at cancer services. I would like to get your e-mail addresses so we can send you guys our newsletter." What the hell? A newsletter! You've got to be kidding me. It was official; I was, literally, the only young person in the room. Was I the only young person in this city with breast cancer? It certainly seemed that way.

Lifting Weights

I tried to separate my personal life from my professional life as much as possible, but breast cancer always found its way into the forefront of my mind all the time. Early one Monday morning, for example, I quickly entered my office building and made a beeline for my office door. As I fumbled with my keys, my assistant, Knekole, stuck her head out of her office and said, "You need some help?"

"No, I got it; thank you," I mumbled. I was trying to avoid her because I didn't want her to see my puffy eyes and ask me why I'd been crying. You see, I never mentioned my breast cancer diagnosis to my team at work. Well, actually, I told one person: Maretta, my lead investigator. She would have to take over while I was out of commission for a while. I trusted Maretta. She has a calm, insightful presence that was very helpful to me during my breast cancer experience. I forbade her to talk to anyone else, though; I wasn't ready for the team to know. I wasn't ready to respond to all the different reactions, emotions, and questions that were sure to follow such an announcement.

As I struggled to open the door, I dropped my keys. Knekole came out of her office, picked up my keys, and opened the door for me. I laughed loudly, trying to distract her from seeing my face. The laughter was weird and unnatural and very awkward. Knekole looked at me as if she was thinking, What the hell is wrong with her? I cleared my throat and rushed into my office, closing the door behind me. As I sat at my desk and stared at the wall, I said to myself, Brianne, you've got relax. Stop being so spastic; you're freaking everybody out.

Knekole knocked on my door and stuck her head in, and said, "So what's on the agenda for today?"

I stared at the computer screen to avoid looking at her and said, "Nothing. I mean reports and everything else."

"What?" she asked.

I took a deep breath and said, "Just do your reports for now, please."

"OK," she responded, looking at me as if I had two heads. "Look, I don't know what's wrong with you, but if you need to talk, I'm here."

"Thank you," I replied. I'm fine." Then she left my office. I reached under my desk and pulled out a book that I had received from my cousin. It was a book of breast cancer survivors' artistic expressions. There were photographs of paintings and sculptures, and there was poetry—different interpretations of their breast cancer experiences. I was in awe of how creative some of these women were. There were also many photographs of women with one breast and some with no breasts at all; they looked so strong. There was a sense of pride in their facial expressions that I could not yet relate to. I wondered if I would ever find a way to artistically interpret my own breast-cancer experience. Would I paint? Would I write? Nope. None of the above. I decided I'd keep my emotions internalized forever. I was not ready to be a part of that club. The breast cancer-members-only club, huh? Thanks, but no thanks.

Knekole burst through my office door as if the building was on fire and quickly took a seat in front my desk. "What's wrong with you? I can hear you sniffing," she said.

"I wasn't sniffing," I said.

"Yes, you were. I'm worried about you; something is definitely wrong with you." Then she looked down at the breast cancer book on my desk.

"First of all, don't come busting in my office all unannounced and uninvited. You'll get a cap bust in your azz doing that." She laughed. "Second of all," I continued, "when I'm ready to talk, I will, OK?"

"OK," she muttered.

As she was walking out, I realized that I actually *was* ready to talk. I'm a Gemini—that's what we do. We talk. I wanted to talk. I wanted to be vocal. I wanted my voice back. "I have breast cancer," I said.

Knekole stopped dead in her tracks, turned around to face me, and said, "Oh no." I nodded in reassurance. "I'm so sorry."

I nodded again. "Thank you." I gave her the whole spiel and brought her up to date; she cried; I cried, and we hugged it out. I could tell her emotions were genuine, and I appreciated her concern for me. I asked her not to tell anyone else; she promised she wouldn't. She hugged me again tightly—really tightly—not as an employee but as a friend. Then I realized how good I felt sharing my diagnosis with her. It really was OK to talk about it, I guessed. I felt like weights were lifting off of me.

My baby, My Hero

One beautiful Saturday morning, I was driving down the street with my babies in the backseat. My mastectomy was only a few weeks away. I was on my way to the store to get some organic gummy bears for the kids. Ever since I was diagnosed with breast cancer, I refused to feed my babies anything with artificial colors since I learned that artificial colors were known carcinogens. As I approached a red light, I looked up into my rearview mirror, and I watched my babies as they played; they were so funny and goofy. I smiled as I watched their beautiful faces. They are the reason I became so depressed during my diagnosis. I became so depressed because of the thoughts I had regarding my children. As a mother, my job was to protect them and nurture them. How could I do that if I was not here? My mind wandered, and I felt a tear roll down my cheek. I could not bear the thought of my babies being without me. Before I knew it, the pain of that possibility completely overwhelmed me again. The tears were flowing without end; I could hardly see. I pulled over to the side of the road to collect myself and calm down. Rhylei, in her usual intelligent, inquisitive demeanor, said, "Mommy, why are you crying?"

I wiped my face and said, "Mommy is just a little sad, baby, but I'm OK."

Rhylei was quiet as she contemplated what I just said; then she said to me, "Mommies don't cry. Babies cry."

Those words resonated in my soul. Those words gave me life in that moment. Those words gave me perspective, strength, and courage. Mommies don't cry, babies cry. "That's right, sweetheart." And it was in that very moment that my attention shifted from a "woe is me" mentality to an "I need to live my life" mentality. Not only was I tired of being sad and worrying but also of obsessing over the unknown. I realized that I could die from anything, any day. Hell, I could walk out of my house tomorrow and get hit by a car. I didn't obsess about potentially getting hit by a car, did I? There was no logic in obsessing over potentially dying from breast cancer. Potentially. Nothing is certain. A new line of questioning began flooding through my mind: How could I live my life *with* this diagnosis? How could I show my babies how much I love them every day? How could I reclaim my voice? My badazzness? I wanted my power back, dammit, and I was determined to get it.

Let's Do This

In the next few days leading up to my mastectomy, I felt stronger and stronger in my will to live. My new motto was "Let's get this shit over with so I can get back to my life." Was I still afraid? Yes. But this time I taught myself how to push past the fear. Prior to my diagnosis, I would speak words of encouragement about entrepreneurship. Entrepreneurship can be scary as hell. Most often, new entrepreneurs would ask me how I became so fearless. I would always tell them, "Being fearless does not mean you are not afraid; it means you accept the fear, and you move forward anyway." That was the advice I gave to others, and now it was time for me to take my own advice. I wrote that statement down on two index cards and taped one on my bathroom mirror above my sink so I could read it every morning to affirm that belief. I also taped one on my refrigerator door. I read it over and over and over again until I actually felt fearless in my breast cancer journey. Punk azz cancer snuck up on me and took my power; I was ready to take it back. I slowly started putting my life into perspective based on facts, not fear. I started realizing the importance of today rather than stressing over tomorrow. I taught myself to live in the present—I mean *really live* in the present. I prioritized my life and gave my attention only to things that really mattered. I eliminated the mind frenzy I was in prior to my diagnosis. I put my phone down and got on the floor with my babies more. I ate better. I exercised more. I gave myself permission to live, to be happy, and to be powerful.

I was in my presurgery room with my mom and hubby in preparation for my second breast cancer surgery. I was about to have a mastectomy. I was nervous, but I wasn't afraid. My husband sensed my nervousness. He walked over to my bed with his cell phone.

"Not Lil Boosie again," I said.

He laughed. "No, just lil Rhylei and lil Rhoey." Then he pulled up pictures and videos of our babies on his phone for me to watch to take my mind off the surgery. He knew that that would make me smile, and it did. In that moment, I felt like I had my support system in the room with me: my mom, my husband, and now my babies were in the room too. Soon the nurse came in to wheel me into surgery.

"Let's do this," I said as they pushed me out of the room.

"We love you! You'll be fine!" Roman and Mom yelled as I left the room. I held a thumbs-up high in the air as I left the room, assuring them I was OK.

I woke up from surgery to a pain I'd never felt before. I needed more medicine. The nurse instructed me to push a button they had placed in my hands so I could self-medicate. In moments, I felt relieved. I looked down at my bandaged chest and thought, Oh my God, my boob is gone. Then I reminded myself that that very same boob had tried to kill me—it needed to go. No tears this time, just hunger. Can I get some food? Where's my husband? When can I go home? I was ready to get out of there—ready to get out of the bandages and get on with my life.

I recovered from my mastectomy at my mom's house so she could help me with the babies. I had a five-pound weight restriction due to the mastectomy, and my babies were each well over twenty-five pounds. It was difficult not being able to pick up my babies for months. They didn't understand why Mommy couldn't hold them. The assistance I received from my mom, dad, and sister during this time was invaluable; they took care of the kids and cooked for us every day. I'm so grateful for them. My family is amazing.

A few days after surgery, it was time for me to shower. I had a drain hanging off my body that was collecting fluid from inside my breast. It was pretty gross. I wondered how I would shower with that contraption hanging off of me. I walked into the bathroom and took my clothes off. I stood there staring into the mirror for a while, looking at the image of myself wearing only underwear and bandages. Wow, one real boob and one fake boob, huh? I thought. I smiled as I remembered my husband saying one real boob and one fake boob were OK with him because now he would have the best of both worlds (lol...men). OK, now let's get these bandages off and see what it looks like. I started taking the bandages off slowly and carefully, noticing how much more bloody they became the closer I got to the wound. Ew, gross, I thought. When the last bandage came off, not only did it reveal my boob, it also revealed the old terrified me. Tears stung my eyes. My boob looked horrible. It was swollen and all stitched up. I closed my eyes, took a deep breath, and reminded myself that this was only the beginning of the reconstruction process, and this was not how it would look in the end. I took a deep breath again, opened my eyes, stared at my boob in the mirror, and said, "I shall call you Frankenboob." Then I laughed at myself and hopped into the shower.

What's important is that I allowed myself to feel the fear as it completely engulfed my body, but this time, panic did not set in. This time, I received the fear, acknowledged it, and immediately released it. This is an important step in reclaiming your power.

Three long months. I had to recover for three long months, and three months seemed like an eternity to me. I continued to run my business from my bed: planning, scheduling, organizing, and delegating. I got constant reminders from everybody to take it easy. I found that increasingly difficult to do. Here I was, stuck in bed, yet my mind was definitely in overdrive—strategizing, setting goals. I was determined to get my voice back. I would not be silenced by this experience. Punk Azz Cancer would not win. As my determination and my mind-set changed, I felt my power grow. As my power grew, the more I felt I needed to get the hell out of that bed. I drove everyone insane because I could not keep still. Here's how Maretta recalls her experience with me during this time:

Brianne the Warrior, by Maretta McDonald

Let's talk about a warrior. *Merriam-Webster* defines a warrior as a person who fights battles and is known for having courage and skill. There's no better word to describe Brianne Sly Fox Joseph. I have been an employee of her private investigation firm for over two years, and I have witnessed a lot of the battles she won and how skillfully she conquered the enemy. No battle was as great as her battle with cancer. This was the battle where she displayed the most courage and skill. From my vantage point, her main weapon was her determination. However, there were times when her determination was bigger than her physical ability. There are a couple of examples that stick out to me more than the rest, and there are quite a few.

Brianne was scheduled for surgery, and I kept in touch with her family regarding her status. They informed me that she was going into surgery, after which I was sitting at home praying and waiting for an update. Later that night, after I had fallen asleep, my mobile phone rang. It was Brianne's number. In my semiconscious state, I immediately panicked, assuming something bad had happened and her family was calling me.

I answered the phone, and I heard a weak, raspy voice on the other line saying, "Maretta, talk to Roman. I need you to..." Then the voice faded, and her husband came on the line. I heard her trying to explain something in the background for him to convey to me. She was trying to ask about my availability to work a case. At that moment I lost my temper but luckily not my job. I went off! I started to fuss angrily into the phone. "Why is she working right now? She just got out of surgery! This is a major surgery! What is she doing? Why is she calling me?"

Her husband, in a very frustrated tone, said, "I know, Maretta; I know." At that moment I realized that the more I argued, the longer she would be talking and not resting. I told him that I would do anything she needed, and we hung up. Brianne had just come out of surgery for mastectomy, not a biopsy or a toenail removal. As angry as I was that she was not concentrating on her recovery, I understood that she was determined to win the battle against this disease and not allow it to disrupt her business.

However, when I thought it couldn't get any worse, it did. There was a child custody case that the agency was working during this time, and the client called with a tip that would provide us an excellent opportunity to gather evidence. The subject of the investigation was at a local bar—this presented a prime opportunity to surveil a person's habits. During this time, the investigators were spread a little thin because our leader was out on injured reserve. Brianne, who was less than a week out of the hospital after the aforementioned surgery, came up with a grand idea that she would work the case.

Let me explain why this was a problem. First, Brianne could not drive due to the surgery; in fact, she couldn't use the arm on that side yet. Second, she still had drains and all of the fresh-out-of-surgery accessories on her. But determination...she had that in abundance. Brianne had her husband drive her to the bar, and she barked instructions on where to park and how to set up for surveillance, like he was her apprentice. Many people may read this and think, "Well, she didn't drive. All she did was sit in the vehicle. It's not that bad." This may be true if that was all that happened.

Against the protest of her driver/husband, she jumped out of the vehicle, hobbling into the bar looking for the subject. She found him and then recorded covert video footage of his activities even though her arm was anchored at her side. I had been communicating with her the entire time by phone while I was trying to get to the location. I reached the location to relieve her in time and watch her gingerly walk back to the vehicle (obviously experiencing some discomfort). All I could do was shake my head in amazement.

Sharing these experiences is not intended to encourage others to do these totally unsafe and crazy things. But they are testimonials of Brianne's warrior spirit. From our conversations throughout the last two years, I learned that she has had to fight for everything that she achieved to date: from her battle to become an African American private investigator to the battles to grow her family businesses. Brianne summoned that spirit in the battle with breast cancer and walked off the battlefield victorious.

Maretta (Sassy Fox) McDonald
Licensed Private Investigator
Sly Fox Investigator

I pretty much drove everyone insane. My desire to live and get back to life became so intense that I was obsessed with planning what I would do as soon as I could get out of bed. Breast cancer had taught me just how precious life was, and I didn't want to waste another second in bed.

Still Entrepreneurial

So, what does an entrepreneurial mind do with idle time? It creates. I was on the Internet one day searching for a breast cancer awareness T-shirt to purchase. I couldn't find anything I liked, so I grabbed a pencil and drew a picture of the type of shirt I wanted to wear. After my mastectomy, I was feeling weak and unattractive. I was embarrassed by my scars. I felt ugly. I wanted to feel beautiful, fearless, and strong again, so I created images of beautiful women who had just returned from war. I created several drawings of these strong, brave women—all different nationalities representing all my sisters around the world who join me daily in this fight against breast cancer. Some had lost their hair; others had not. I called them the "Anaba Alliance." *Anaba* is a word that means "she returns from war." I recalled the pain that I felt the day my mother pulled the covers off my face and made me get out of bed when I was depressed. As I arose from my bed, in disgust I had mumbled, "Punk azz cancer," realizing how cancer had tried to take me away from my family. That's what I decided to name my new business: Punk Azz Cancer (punkazzcancer.com). That was the day I reconnected with my power. It was the day I became a member of the Anaba Alliance.

Prior to my breast cancer diagnosis, my husband and I also owned a tattoo shop. Our experience with breast cancer inspired us to collaborate and create Body of Art—a paramedical-services center. Women like me who have had a mastectomy are often left with scars or without a nipple and areola. I knew firsthand how that image affected a woman's self-esteem. Our company, Body of Art, tattoos realistic, 3-D nipples and tattoos on women who have undergone a mastectomy. The results are invaluable because not only do we restore the nipple, we also restore the woman's confidence.

I didn't find a lot of resources in my area for young breast cancer survivors, so I also became the state leader for the Young Survival Coalition, which is an organization that provides breast-cancer resources to women under forty.

Early detection saved my life, and I was determined to bring awareness to that fact in hopes of saving the lives of other young women. Determination is a powerful force. Having a strong sense of determination is vital to your survival and vital to your path to reclaiming your power. And I don't mean just any old "average" form of determination. I mean having laser sharp focus on obtaining your goal of reclaiming your power. You must develop a *burning desire* to reclaim your power- a desire so intense that you absolutely refuse to be defeated. Let me give you an example of the type of determination I'm referring to: I created my t-shirt line only two weeks after having my mastectomy. Only two weeks! And this book was written in only a few months after my mastectomy. It was written *while* I was completing my breast reconstruction. That's how determined I was to continue my path as an entrepreneur. I decided that nothing would take that away from me- not even breast cancer. That is the same type of determination you need to reach your goals- any goals you may have, not just regarding breast cancer. When you are determined to rise, you will. It's inevitable my friends. I did it, and you can as well.

What is power?

This life is yours. Take the power to choose what you want to do and do it well. Take the power to love what you want in life and love it honestly. Take the power to control your own life. No one else can do it for you. Take the power to make your life happy.

—Susan Polis Schultz

Nothing else will shake up your world more than hearing the words, "You have cancer." And if you're reading this, you, yourself, have probably heard those words or something similar, recently. Now you may be looking for answers—not necessarily medically, but perhaps emotionally and mentally. How do you go on? What do you do now? How will you handle this? You may feel afraid, depressed, or defeated.

The dictionary defines power as "a right or authority that is given to or delegated to a person; the ability or right to control."

Power comes in living your life in the midst of your breast cancer journey. It is about finding your happiness in the midst of your struggle. Power is taking control of your thoughts when circumstances are absolutely beyond your control. In the midst of these uncontrollable circumstances, a powerful mind-set can help us direct our lives in a positive direction. In the midst of tragedy, we feel out of control. We feel pain, and we feel sadness. We are surrounded by darkness and despair. We feel hopeless. It's not that we lack power. It is that we lack the awareness of it, and we lack the belief in it. A positive perception of yourself and your circumstances is the first step to realizing your power. Power begins in your mind. When you control your mind, you control your actions. When you control your actions, you control your life. When we tap into our personal power, we learn to become resilient. We learn how to recover from hard times and setbacks. We get knocked down, but we learn how to stand tall. We get up. Every time. When you find your power, you will be unmoved by all the chaos that surrounds you. You'll find courage in the midst of uncertainty. Power is being completely unfazed by the very same things that previously would have forced us to our knees. My dark days gave me a story—they didn't make me powerful. I was already powerful. My dark days made me prove it.

How do you find your power?

Your power is hidden in your mind-set. I had to train my mind in order to change my view of my circumstances. What I found most helpful was the use of positive affirmations. Positive affirmations are carefully crafted sentences that we say to ourselves to encourage a positive attitude. It's no more complex than that, but the power they have is absolutely amazing. A few of the affirmations I used throughout my journey were "I am stronger than fear"; "I am powerful beyond my own belief"; and "I am resilient. I *will* get through this." I repeated these every day until I believed it. We humans are incredible creatures. But in the end, our experience of the world is limited to two things: we have sensory awareness through what we can touch, smell, hear, taste, and see, and we have our attitude toward those sensory experiences. There was a man who lived through the Holocaust and afterward wrote *Man's Search for Meaning*. His name was Viktor E. Frankl. In it he said that everything can be taken from a man except one thing, the last of the human freedoms: that is, to choose one's attitude in any given set of circumstances, to choose one's own way. That man lived through what we cannot fathom, and he didn't have any bit of control over his situation. So what did he do? He created his own control. He controlled his own attitude, and by doing so, he took the power away from those who sought to break him, and he used the power within himself to find the strength to move on.

It's easy when you are going through a difficult situation like breast cancer to lose sense of who you really are. Our identity gets tangled up in the situation we are faced with, and we start to identify only with that situation. I was not in the Holocaust, but like Viktor E. Frankl, I had no control over my situation. I could take the right medicines, and I could do all the right things, but I had no power to control how they would work. All I could do was shape my own attitude.

And I shaped my attitude through the use of affirmations. I said them every morning when I woke up, and I repeated them every time I felt overwhelmed. Affirmations and phrases can definitely help you build your strength. Affirmations can help you think positively and stay on track with your successes, big or small. Repeating affirmations each day will help you stay calm and focused. The sheer power of saying positive words out loud is palpable. You can feel it in your gut. Positive affirmations change our view of the world, and so, for many of us, they can actually change our world in a very positive way.

What is personal inner strength?

Inner strength is defined differently by different people. One of the most common definitions of inner strength is being confident about the power you have inside, having the determination to win, and rising above fear. But how exactly do you do that? To find your inner strength, you should have a clear understanding of what exactly inner strength is and what it means. Is it simply a state of mind? Is it what you think about yourself? Is it what you believe you can do? It is definitely more than just putting words together to create affirmations and phrases. Inner strength is built upon a firm belief in your affirmations. Repeating an affirmation is one thing, but making a declaration regarding your affirmation is totally different. It's all about your mind-set. What do you really believe? Do you really believe you will be OK? The reality is, none of us know what will happen tomorrow. We will never have the ability to predict the future. But does that mean we have to live in fear? Absolutely not. We learn to be fearless so that we can live *today*. Today is all we have. It's all any of us have.

At any given moment, any of us can walk outside and get hit by a car. Do we decide to remain inside our house every day for fear of getting hit by a car? Of course not. Do you see my point? We cannot live in fear of dying from breast cancer. Anyone can die from anything at any time. With that knowledge, we can spend our time better by focusing on living and moving forward. But we will never move forward if we don't acknowledge the fear we face—and let it go. Remember: Fearless does not mean you aren't afraid. It means you accept the fear and move forward anyway. The key is to move forward in spite of the fear. Your courage is waiting on the other side of fear.

To find that courage and inner strength, you'll also need to have inner peace. You are living in a world of chaos. Diagnosis and treatment can happen really fast! You're thrown into the race with little to no information to help you make big decisions very quickly. It's stressful. It's difficult to be strong when you are not at peace within. You will have to find time to be still, to be quiet, to clear your mind, to meditate. You will have to find your center. Power comes in clarity of thought. Once you're able to get a grasp on your situation, once you realize you do have a plan, and once you understand what is required of you to get through this, you'll soon realize that you are, without a doubt, capable of handling this. You will realize that, without a doubt, you can actually survive.

My spiritual beliefs and my faith got me through this difficult time. Everything in this world is has a purpose. The events that transpire in our lives are purposed from beginning to end. There is nothing that we can do to change the outcome of any event. What we can do, however, is control the way we view the situation and the way we handle it. I changed my vocabulary and strove to remove all negativity from it. I strove to remove all the defeatist attitudes that I imposed on myself. I refrained from using sentences such as "I can't" or "That's impossible" or "I can't do this." I made the choice to turn the negative in my life into something positive. You can do the same thing. Even on those days when I felt completely overwhelmed by my own thoughts, I took a step back to regroup and evaluate my thought processes. When I realized I was focusing on the negative, I would immediately change my focus to something positive. Yes, I was given a breast cancer diagnosis, but I'm still here. It's not over. I'm still here. That in and of itself is a true blessing.

You are your biggest support system

You have support from people all around you, but you are the most important support system you will ever need. We all have our dark days. Dark days are inevitable. But once you tap into your personal power, you'll find that your own inner strength will get you through the darkness. Receiving a diagnosis of breast cancer was like having all the lights turned off in my world. I felt as if I was on a dark road with no direction, no map. It wasn't until I changed my mind-set that I was able to come out of the darkness. Your inner strength is that voice deep down inside that says, "I can, and I will," regardless of what the circumstances are and regardless of the hand you are dealt in life. Just as we feed our bodies healthy food for nourishment, we must also feed our minds positive, healthy thoughts as well. Be mindful of what you're telling yourself. Be mindful of your own messages. We believe ourselves more than we will ever believe anyone else. I'm confident that soon you will find the courage and determination to keep persisting. We have everything we need already inside of us to be powerful; it's already there. We just have to learn to tap into that source for strength and guidance. Be fearless, my friends. Live with intention; find your happiness in the midst of your struggle, and—most important—kick azz, and stand in your power.

About The Author

Brianne Joseph, LPI, is an award-winning entrepreneur, author, speaker, and business coach. She is the owner and head investigator at Sly Fox Investigations, a six-figure all-female investigative agency. Brianne as been a licensed private investigator in the state of Louisiana for eleven years. She is a married mother of two. Brianne has written and published articles about private investigation and has been a guest on radio shows as well. A true leader, Mrs. Joseph was previously appointed the region II director of the Louisiana Private Investigators Association. In addition, this innovative investigator was named the 2011 Investigator of the Year by the National Association of Investigative Specialists. She has been featured in several local and national publications, including the *Baton Rouge Business Report*, *225* magazine, the *Louisiana Weekly*, the *Atlanta Post*, *Essence* magazine, and many others. Mrs. Joseph was also honored at the Baton Rouge Professionals 40 under 40 Entrepreneurs Award ceremony.

As a sought after speaker, Brianne is a crowd favorite and enjoys speaking about entrepreneurship as well as being resilient and driven in spite of difficult circumstances. She has recovered from losing everything in 2005 during Hurricane Katrina and again in 2016 during the great flood of Louisiana. As a breast cancer survivor, she inspires other victims with her personal story of turning tragedy to triumph through her Punk Azz Cancer empowerment brand. Her mission is to teach others how to turn their pain into power, just as she has done throughout her life. She is also an advocate for young breast cancer survivors as the State Leader for the Young Survival Coalition. Brianne also enjoys coaching aspiring entrepreneurs.

She has been a volunteer counselor and community presenter for the Capital Area Family Violence Intervention

Center (CAFVIC) Battered Women's shelter and has also spoken to our community's younger generations about having confidence and knowing their self worth.

Learn more about Brianne at

www.slyfoxinvestigations.com

briannejoseph.com

punkazzcancer.com

Phone: 225-305-7468

For Speaking engagements,

E-mail: slyfox@slyfoxinvestigations.com

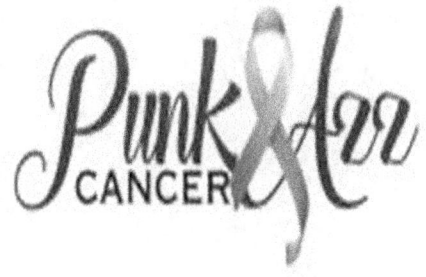

Visit punkazzcancer.com for Breast Cancer
resources and Anaba Alliance merchandise and apparel.

www.ingramcontent.com/pod-product-compliance
Lightning Source LLC
Chambersburg PA
CBHW070225290526
45789CB00004B/1520